READY TO TAKE ACTION

Marcus Sassi

Ready to Take Action

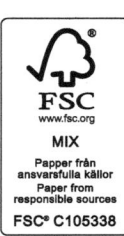

Photo: **Catalin Ionescu / caiofoto.se**
Translation: **Marcus Sassi**
Additional contributor: **Mia Sassi**

Publishing and printing: BoD

ISBN: 978-91-7463-582-9

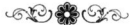

This book is dedicated to my father,
Charles Sassi.
I will forever love you.

- Your son, Marcus

Table of Contents

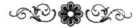

Acknowledgements

I would like to thank God for everything in life. There are no words that can really describe everything that I feel, but I want to say that I'm grateful for everything.

Secondly, I want to thank my wife, Mia Sassi, for all her loving support over the years. I couldn't have done this without you. You have always been there for me, no matter the circumstances. I am grateful for everything you have done and said, and for you allowing me be a part of your life; I thank God that our roads crossed. We were young when we met, I loved you back then, I love you now, and I will always love you.

To my daughter, Leona, Mum and Dad love you so much. I thank God every day for blessing your mother and me with you. The love we have for you can't be measured.

I want to thank my stepmother Nicole, my father Charles, brother Drolin, brother Bob, sister Jennifer, and sister Yvictorie, my aunt Marie, and her husband Kams.

Also, thanks to the children, Juislaine, Samuel, Adelinee, and Vanessa.

Big thanks to Raul Garcia for the tremendous amount of work you put in on marcussassi.com. I am amazed and blown away at the same time. I want to thank everyone on my staff at marcussassi.com for everything you have done; you guys have really walked the extra miles to make this dream become a reality – we did it!

Thanks also goes to my friends Mustafa Iskandar, Kevan Issa, Christopher Pecanac, Ali Coaney, Haroun Hajem, Catalin Ionescu, Mohamud Salad, Mustafa Ahmed, Malick Bah, and Nur Abdulle for believing in me and motivating me. Thank you.

How to best use this book

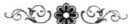

In order to achieve the highest level of development, we recommend that the reader use this book along with the action planner and the other tools provided at marcussassi.com We believe that this book will provide you with the foundation needed for your growth, the action planner will provide you with the practical training, and marcussassi. com can be your resource database that is continually updated with tools to elevate you to greatness. We recommend that you read straight through from the first chapter to the last chapter, but it's not necessary if you don't want to. Remember, it's your path – you choose it!

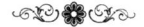

Chapter 1

What made me

I couldn't stop crying, the pain was too
much. What was I supposed to do now and
what would I tell my father, I wondered as I
sat there crying on the kitchen floor. I heard
every word she said but I was too devastated.
I was finished and I couldn't take it anymore.

A voice in my head told me that I had to
follow through and that letting go was not
an option. I was silent for a moment as I
pulled myself together. She was still there, so
I reached for the phone and confirmed that
I was ready to go on now. She said that there
was nothing else to do – I had reached the
end of the line.

She was a debt collector.

The days were always warm in the home country of Congo-Kinshasa. We lived in a large house with a plot of just over 21,000 sq. ft., with a large tree in the middle of the plot, where we spent much of our time together –my brother, my aunt, my uncle and I. We used to sit there in the evenings; we ate food and watched the stars together. The fences that surrounded the plot formed a wall approximately 2 meters high. In the daytime, I played with the neighbors' children and in the afternoons, I played with my dog, which my aunt did not know anything about.

The dog was always waiting for me outside, as if it knew that our friendship had to be preserved as a secret. It was also with me at home on the farm when no one was around. It was a Doberman – a great friend to which I became much attached to. I feared that my aunt knew about the dog, even though I had not said anything. I would not have been surprised if the neighbors had blabbed to her about it.

My uncle taught me all about agriculture, about how he sowed the seeds of the earth, how to irrigate, and how often it had to be watered. We had a few chickens; poor fellas, they had to run when I chased them. There came a day when my uncle wanted to show me the process of how to kill a chicken and prepare it for cooking. It was a scary thought for me. He asked me to fetch a chicken and I guess that the chicken knew what would happen next, because on that day, it ran as it had never done before. I chased it for at least ten minutes before I got a hold of it. I carried it up to the table where my uncle was and placed it on the table.

My uncle said that it was important that we showed gratitude for the gift we had received – to respect the chicken and thank it for its bounty. He asked me to hold the chicken while he killed it. He took out a small ax and cut its throat; I panicked and dropped the chicken, which meant that I witnessed it running around headless – it was a horrible sight. My uncle was the wise one, while my aunt was the strong one – no one could push her around. I had only seen fear in her eyes once, which was when we went off to apply for visas and papers to travel out of the country, as we had received news from my father, who was in Europe.

He had finally received a residence permit in Sweden, which meant that we could now travel to him. I had no memory of my father, nor any pictures, and did not even know his name. He had moved away before I was born to prepare a better life for us in Europe. I did not know anything about my mother either, but that did not bother me, because I knew how much my aunt loved us. I knew it by the way she used to hug us. When we went to the embassy, I remember sitting in my aunt's arms in the car on the way; there were so many soldiers on the road there and we were stopped many times on the road for inspection. It was a scary sight with all their weapons. My aunt was scared, and I was scared, but at the same time, very calm. My aunt held me so tightly that I knew she never would allow anything to happen to us; it was a very reassuring feeling.

It went well at the embassy, although they were initially reluctant and did not want to cooperate. However, no one says no to my aunt, so it all ended well with the application and we got our papers approved. Every evening, my uncle used to say, "Oh boys, now you're going to your father in Europe. After you have been there for a while, you will begin to change. You will become white like the people who live there."

I was very excited to meet my father; every night was spent on the farm under the tree. I often looked at the moon and thought of my father. I simply could not wait. Then came the day that we were to travel; I do not remember the trip to the airport, but soon, the plane was on the way to Germany. I could not hold back any longer; I was so excited that I told everyone who would listen that I was going to meet my Dad. I think everyone on the plane knew my family history with how loud I was talking. I was a short and skinny little boy with a big belly, like what older men usually have.

I held my aunt's hand very tight when we stepped off the plane in Sweden. I did not know who my father was, so I trusted blindly that my aunt would recognize him. She walked up to a man and hugged him and I could tell that she was so happy. I remember that she had the world's biggest smile; she was clearly hugging my father. This was to become the best day of my life.

The first city in Sweden that I lived in was Uddevalla, but that was only for a year. We later moved to a larger city. I did not recall seeing any other immigrants beside our family and the families of my father's friends. My first friends in Sweden were Adam and Madeleine; I remember that everyone used to tease us, "There goes Marcus and Madde."

The first day Adam and Madde had approached me, I knew no words in Swedish, but somehow we communicated and gradually became good friends. Uddevalla was where I learned to ride a bicycle and where I saw snow for the first time; it was amazing to see it fall from the sky and turn the landscape white. My father told us that the key to growth in any country is strong language skills, so he said that no one besides him and my aunt were to speak other languages than Swedish. At first, I thought that was weird, because the first week we barely spoke, since we knew nothing in Swedish. However, thanks to practicing at home and listening to Adam and Madeleine, we eventually started to speak Swedish.

I will never forget the day my father brought me to town for the very first time. The reason for that powerful memory is that the whole town froze. Everyone stopped whatever he or she was doing to stare at my father and me. Heads turned when we passed by and I felt horrible with how they looked at us. I gripped my father's hand hard and he looked at me. I did not say a word, but he knew what I was thinking: *Please Dad, let's hurry out of here.* That was the first time I felt that I was far from home and not welcome. I was crying on the inside. Later that day, I showered for over an hour, thinking about what my uncle had told us: that we would eventually turn into white people. I tried hard to wash away my skin color, because I did not want to be so different from everyone else.

I did not want to go through what I had just experienced ever again. I did not leave home for a few days. I just lay in bed, crying silently so no one would hear me.

A year passed, and it was time to move to Bergsjön, which is on the outskirts of the city of Gothenburg, a beautiful place with nature all around. As a young African, there were at that time no role models or people with whom I could identify, aside from my father and stepmother. I never saw an African in the workforce, none in the cafés, banking, housing, or any other marketplace. It was tough growing up in Bergsjön. I remember when my elementary school teacher told me that I needed to make sure to push myself in life if I were to have a chance at anything, and that I needed to be at least ten times better than the native Swedes in order to be accepted in their society.

Her message stuck with me and is something I have carried with me ever since. My life became dedicated to doing everything in my power to help my father and to prove how wrong other people's preconceived beliefs truly were. The climate was raw in our neighborhood; there were no footsteps to imitate, but I was not the only one that felt like this. The rhetoric that flourished during that time was that people who grew up in that neighborhood had a high likelihood of falling into crime and alienation.

Many young people felt this, and their frustration was taken out on each other. I remember kids coming from other parts of the neighborhood just to pick a fight. I understand that now; they had no recreational activities and nothing to relate to, nothing to which they could attach themselves. Unemployment was very high in the area where I grew up.

Luckily, being aware of my father's struggle and commitment made me turn my life around and I was grateful for that. Many others that I grew up with turned into juvenile delinquents. Some did actually turn their lives around, but that was much later in life.

I was grateful for the work of my father and his siblings; they had to make sacrifices so that we could get to Sweden and have a chance at a better life. Knowing this gave me strength and determination to make a real effort in school and focus on making the best of my leisure time. It was not easy, but I always tried.

I remember an elderly woman on my way to school that was collecting cans from trash bins, which she later took to the grocery store for some money in exchange. It confirmed to me that her life was not the way I was going to end up. I respected her, because who am I to judge anyone, not knowing her story, but I could see the pain in her. My process of growing up was about refuting the idea of being alienated or having the tendency to be a criminal; I was not one of the lost souls that they tried to depict.

Wherever we went, people were afraid when they heard about where we came from. Many times, I was rejected from jobs because of the area in which I resided. My primary and middle school teachers saw potential in me and motivated me to spend extra time on my studies. I liked going to school, learning new things, and being challenged. My father always wanted what was best for us, and when I turned thirteen, I was sent to a school located on the other side of the city. He wanted a school that had few students with foreign background so I would have a greater chance of interacting with the natives and improving my language skills. The school was far away and none of my friends studied nearby; all of my friends studied in Bergsjön. I was the only one who had to commute to school, so going to a school in a neighborhood that I was not familiar with was tough at times.

I did come to like my new school and my classmates, many of whom I'm still friends with today. However, I did start to slip away from some of my old friends; we were still friends, but we saw each other less frequently.

Years later, I lost contact with them, which is sad, as some were truly good people.

The thought of being a minority, of being a black man in Europe raised in Bergsjön, practically doomed me to a hard life, and it was always in the back of my mind. I wanted to disprove their preconceived beliefs; I wanted to show that you could make it if you committed yourself. My inspiration was my father; he had moved to a country he knew nothing about, yet now, we had shelter over our heads and food on the table. For me, that was a great achievement.

I wanted to be a role model for young people; I wanted to create a path that they could follow, in order to make it easier for even more people. I became interested in entrepreneurship and created a record label with a childhood friend. We were young just 17 years old with ambitions to take over the music world, and it actually went so well that we even took on a trainee. We sold no goods, but we had created a name for ourselves. Many people had high expectations for us, so we entered into a partnership with a recreation center that I also helped to build; I was also a member of its board. The goal was to produce a CD that gathered the city's most talented and influential artists. The news had spread about the business and we started receiving demos from all corners of Sweden, Denmark, and Norway – artists who wanted to sign a record contract with us.

The project with the compilation CD was sent out to the printers and we printed a lot of CDs, but we had to cancel when we heard the news that one of the artists had used copyrighted material without permission, which made people fear a lawsuit against our label and the recreation center. The board decided that we could no longer go on with the project; the partnership had to end. Our future was depending on the release of the compilation CD, people expected the CD, and yet I had to go to the marketplace and inform everyone that we had cancelled the project. Our business took a major hit, and we lost whatever credibility we had.

Our reputation was down to zero, and everyone in town, as well as people in Denmark and Norway, knew about this. I couldn't go anywhere without people recognizing me, talking, and pointing fingers, saying, "There goes the record label manager that failed everyone." We eventually terminated the business.

I had failed, but that was not going to be the end of me.

Even though it hurts to think about it, how am I supposed to not love him? Looking back, everything played out just as I had wished for. My wife even mistook me for him when she looked at a photo of me. I had become my father, the man that loved me and hurt me at the same time. I understand now that he had no choice; he couldn't afford being absent from work. He didn't have to say much; by looking in his eyes, you could simply tell the sacrifice and commitment he had to uphold so that my siblings and I could have the foundation he had provided. I cherished his will power, for I had my mind made up that one day I would be able to provide for him, just has he had done for me.

What hurts me the most was not having an absent father; I could handle not having him visit me during my soccer games, never have him see my projects, or the businesses I ran – I could handle it. However, what hurts me the most was seeing my father take on jobs that were below his qualifications. I didn't like seeing the amount of hours he had to work, or seeing him grow older because of the hard labor. That is what hurt me the most.

My father used to be a math teacher back in Congo-Kin-shasa, but now worked as a taxi driver in a new country far from home. He always put on a smile, but I knew him better than that; I could see how much he actually suffered.

My father, my hero, gave me the best gift of all without even knowing it. I was able to feel his pain and his hunger for a better life for his family. He had become my reason to fight.

Chapter 2

You are capable of more

A major contributing factor for my capacity to move forward is the faith of my own characteristics, the belief that I am capable of so much more than meets the eye, and the knowledge that no obstacles are insurmountable. This way of thinking has helped me and I strongly believe it can help you too. Therefore, I recommend that you choose to invest in yourself. I often say to my friends and to myself, "*You know more than you think. You have abilities and capabilities that only you have. Some things can only be carried out by you and no one else, so don't stop investing in yourself.*"

In my businesses, my focus has always been on developing my staff. I try to find out where their true passions lie and then I invest in their training or provide tools that will strengthen and develop their capacity. I also work to create an environment where they feel comfortable and feel that they have the ability to influence and develop. My ideology has always been to look out and care for my employees. If I do that, they will in turn take care of the business.

It has not always been easy and I guess it won't ever be; every new group will bring new challenges, but I'm getting better at it. I didn't succeed the first time, but it is a strategy that I have come to understand as being aligned with my own belief. It is extremely satisfying to see people find their inner glow and see how much happier and more productive they become in their job. I love helping people reach their full potential, and as I mentioned before, I didn't succeed the first time. I have failed many times, but I decided to get back up and try again. Every time, the end results keep getting better and better.

I think hanging on and not seeing failure as a failure, but rather as feedback, has also been a contributing factor to my success. Every new piece of feedback takes me back to the drawing board and I get to study what happened, why it happened, what factors drove us to the failure, and what could be done differently next time. Then, I try again.

Believing in oneself, no matter what life situation occurs, requires mental strength. Don't listen to the negative inner voices that tell you that you can't do it. Instead, we should spend our time doing something else, such as going back to our comfort zone.

I believe that as you move toward greater success, love, abundance, and creativity in your life, you will encounter an obstacle, a self-belief obstacle, but that new challenge brings a priceless gift hidden within it. The gift will reveal itself as you explore and overcome the obstacle. The gift itself is a special relationship with your inner sparkle. The obstacle is actually a limit that we have all placed on ourselves, and it's essential for your growth that you overcome this obstacle if you are to enjoy everything that life has to offer. This limitation is often present when we get a bit older and start to live with the awareness of societal structures. When we dream about achieving major goals, we often talk ourselves out of pursuing that goal or dream.

If we don't overcome these self-hindering beliefs, we'll always talk ourselves out of the opportunities that come our way.

I would never be in the position I am right now if I had allowed the negative inner voice to lead me away from pursuing my life dream of empowering people, helping them overcome their obstacles, and moving them toward reaching their full potential. The first step I had to take was to overcome the belief that I was not capable, that because of my current environment, my African heritage, or my immigrant status, I couldn't move into higher realms.

I've met people who have done great things and who seek to achieve even greater things in life that started off with a great attitude, but when things went their way, they backed off. They actually did everything in their power to neglect the success, as if they were not worthy of it, because great things were not supposed to happen to them – they faced a fear of success.

One thing that I struggled with for a long time was self-guilt. I felt guilty for pursuing my dreams because it meant I would need to change my environment and change the people I spent most of my time with – I faced the fear of change with guilt of being disloyal toward my friends. My mind said, *Who do you think you are going for you dreams, Superman or something?* Yet at the same time, I felt a strong urge to pursue my dreams because if I succeeded, my friends would succeed too. However, it took me many years to overcome those thoughts.

I gathered some old friends and one by one I told them that I would be absent for some time. I told them that I wasn't sure when we would see each other again and that I needed to devote my life to pursuing my dreams. Some of them supported me and some thought I was acting weird and stupid; one of them even said that I would never amount to anything, and that I would go nowhere.

I am actually glad that happened, because at least I got a confirmation of who believed in me and who did not.

Self-belief is so important, so I hope that after you've read this chapter, it will come to be just as important for you. I feel that many of us tend to run away from our true essence and our true nature due to a lack of self-belief. We need to believe the fact that all of us are unique and that there will never be another like you. I strongly believe that if people would begin to believe in themselves, they would find strength, resources, and capabilities that they never knew they had.

That reminds me of the time I wanted to take a math course. I was working at that time and my employer had granted me a couple of hours to attend the introduction meeting. The students had to do a math test to see whether they had a strong enough math background to be able to pass the course. I did not do well at all and the teacher told me that he did not want to accept me into the course because of the exam results. He said that I would not make it, that the course was too advanced - above my knowledge. I told him that I would succeed in the course, and that it did not matter what he said – I would make it. I told him that it was written in the stars that I would succeed.

We had a short argument, but eventually he gave in, saying not to blame him, that my success or failure was on me. I got back to work and my supervisor asked me how the exam went. I told her that it went horrible, but that it did not matter, because I would succeed in the course. I asked if I could take two weeks of vacation, as I needed to focus on the course, and she granted my request.

Later that same day, I told my present wife, although we were not married at that time. I told her that for the coming two weeks, I needed to be by myself. I was going to lock myself in the home office for two weeks and study. She was very supportive and even got me a blackboard that we hung on the wall. I only left the room to use the bathroom or at mealtimes.

I decided that I would prove my teacher wrong; not doing well on that exam, did not determine my future. I was committed to achieving my goal. I studied every day from early morning until late in the evening. When I got tired, I told myself, *Don't you give up on me now; you can do one more hour.* I had to talk myself into pushing forward. That inner voice did everything to stop me. It told me that I was tired, that I should take a break, go to bed and get some sleep, or watch TV. It tried all kind of things to get me out of that room and I fought it every time; I told myself, *No, you are not quitting now. You shall continue. It does not matter how tough it is, you are going to do it.*

Two weeks passed and it was time for the next exam. I went to school and took the exam. The teacher called me later that day, telling me that he had gone through the exam and was amazed by my results. He wanted to congratulate me personally on successfully executing the exam and that math was definitely "my thing." He also said that he was very proud of me.

As you read this, I want you to know that you should not hold back from expressing the full potential of your inner greatness. When we don't limit ourselves, it liberates great potential that will draw us to new heights of greatness. Looking back, I'm more than grateful for stepping forwards toward my dreams.

My message to you:

1. Have faith in your own abilities.
2. Believe that you are more than meets the eye.
3. You know more than you think.
4. There are abilities and capabilities that only you have.
5. Some things can only be carried out by you and no one else.
6. Do only things that are aligned with your core beliefs.
7. Believe that no obstacle is insurmountable.
8. Invest in your own training.
9. Never give up.
10. Learn from your previous mistakes.
11. Do not listen to naysayers.
12. You do not need to fit in; be yourself, be weird.
13. You deserve all the success you aim for.

Chapter 3
Mental growth & self-image

For me, mental training and mental strength
is the ability to maintain a constant positive
outlook, particularly in terms of your own
abilities. My hope is that after reading the
previous chapter, you will have begun believing in yourself and in your own abilities.
Mental strength is about developing the ability to have a constant positive attitude. It's
not easy, however, and it is something you
need to work on throughout your life, for we
constantly face forces that want to put us out
of balance. Therefore, we need to keep ourselves strong, no matter what we encounter
in life.

We need to stay strong when things do not go our way, or when we encounter negative forces that wish to set us on a negative path or in a negative mindset.

This reminds of the time I was being bullied at work by my coworkers. They disliked me because I did not share their beliefs. All they spoke about was, according to me, filthy talk. They said all kinds of nasty things about other coworkers, the leaders, and the business in general. I felt that what they were doing was not something that was aligned with my beliefs, so I was bullied. They even sang songs about me and did all kinds of nasty things. However, I knew in my mind that attacking other people was a sign of weakness, which I did not do, so I was winning. I also knew in my mind that all they wanted was to get inside my head and get a reaction from me, which would only feed them to continue bullying me.

It went on for a very long time, and I did not speak with anyone about it. I knew that they were waiting for a response and that I should remain calm, rather than let outer forces control me, and I did everything in my power to not think about it and continue life like nothing was happening. I had to fill my mind up with other thoughts – positive thoughts. The bullying increased for some time, which was an indication that they were getting frustrated and desperate. I just needed to continue on the path I had chosen. They eventually stopped and gave up – they could not reach me.

A situation like this also occurred at a different job. A colleague of mine was talking to his friends about being short of money and how nice it would be if they were millionaires. I approached them, said that I had overheard their conversation and if he really wanted to be a millionaire, I could stay after my shift and teach him financial management so that he could one day become wealthy. His friends laughed and looked at me like, *'Who is this guy? Who does he think he is?'* My colleague looked down at his desk and then laughed.

I saw that deep down, he wanted my help, but could not go against his friends. I told him that if he ever needed me, he should just let me know and then I left. My message to you is never give up on your dreams, even if everyone else around you says that you cannot succeed.

I started my journey of building mental strength by constantly saying to myself, *"It's possible."* I don't know how many times I said that to myself every day, but after saying it for a while, you will start to believe it. You will start to believe that things are possible for you and that everything depends on how you choose to react to what is happening around you. I stopped believing that only outside factors influenced and got me to act in a certain ways; now, I know that I always have a choice of how to react, so I no longer depend on outside factors – it's all me.

It is certainly true that we become what we think. An example is that when I am interested in starting a new business, I think of how amazing it would be to start the company and achieve the goal. Another person might instead think about how tough it would be, the demands it would place, and the risks it would entail. The end result is that they usually talk themselves out of starting a company that they have always desired. They may start, but only because someone else talked them into it. However, I want to suggest that conviction from within and not from an external impact, will always be stronger.

So how does one change life for the better? I think it all starts from within; it starts from our thoughts. People who take on new paths tend to think differently. It's not just about positive thinking; it's the ability to think properly in different contexts. Decisive factors, according to me, are what you think about and how you choose to direct them in your mind. It is important to develop the ability to think positively about yourself and other people, rather than place any limits on oneself.

A positive person thinks positive thoughts about themselves and others, while a negative person thinks negatively about themselves and others. I usually say that it is important to clean up the brain, which can be done by constantly thinking positively, no matter the circumstances in life. The reason I want you to focus on positive thinking is that the more positively you think, the more positive thoughts will take place in your mind. What happens then is that the brain will struggle to produce negative thoughts. People will come to experience you as a positive force – a person that brings joy. What I have also noticed over the years is that positive people tend to help other people, while negative people refrain from lending a helping hand. Positive people are happy to share. What I do in order to stay positive is to write down the distribution between positive and negative thoughts, particularly the thoughts that have been the most dominant during the day. I then consider how these thoughts affect my life and what I'm willing to do to change my way of thinking so those negative thoughts don't visit me again.

I tend to ask myself how much I have been affected by external forces and how I should have thought differently. The end goal here is to increase awareness, because when you become aware, you suddenly understand that you always have a choice. You can either accept the negative or say "no" to it and instead focus on thinking about something more positive.

Therefore, it is important to reflect, because reflection creates awareness and it is an important ingredient in your development. This has helped me tremendously. Another important aspect of mental strength is the ability to think correctly, which is how you see yourself. How you see yourself creates safety and security that is invaluable in different situations. With a positive self-image, you can have a brand new attitude that reflects in how you dress, speak, walk, and live – even your surroundings will be perceived in a completely different way, all based on how you see yourself.

When I look back at my life and think of all the projects and companies I have started, how some have done better than others, and about all the those times I have had to terminate projects or companies, or how I could have easily given up, it is obvious that I have failed so many times in life that I have given up counting. However, something inside of me always knew that one day I would succeed and that I should never give up, no matter how bad things seemed. Many have asked me why I keep on going, failure after failure, but what they do not understand is that my "why" – my reason to fight – is too strong. How I choose to see myself has been the decisive factor.

How you view yourself is linked to all the memories and experiences in your life, both positive and negative. My experiences and memories have conditioned me to the point of transformation into a person that never accepts that things will always be as they are. I've always thought that things can change and get better and that there is always a solution. Thus, I have worked my way forward, for the danger lies in accepting the way things are. The risk is that a person gets stuck in that belief and eventually stops believing in themselves. Something that I agree with strongly is that hope is the last thing to leave you. By keeping faith in the dream, it will always remain alive.

I hope that after reading this chapter, you can begin to see yourself in a more positive way, as a person that thinks in a positive manner, treats oneself with respect, care, and love. That person is proud of accomplishments, thinks positively, and acts positively, meaning they have no reason to talk negatively or look down on other people. They wish only positive things for themselves and others.

Another thing that has helped me in my journey is putting more energy into developing my positive and negative abilities, constantly developing myself into a better person. This is not just for me, but also for the people around me. I am not afraid to ask for help from those who want to see me succeed. Helping others is a form of mutual growth.

Something that can have a serious effect on self-image is our surroundings. We are constantly bombarded with other people's opinions – what other people think about us, TV, radio, billboards, media, and social media; this can either cause us to grow or diminish us, so it's extremely important that you develop a positive self-image.

I would like to say that besides thinking positively, you also need to have a clear vision of the things you would like to do and the person you would like to be. Mistakes that I often see are when people only try to change their outer self-image – the way they dress, smell, and look. That's great, but the problem is that they do not get long-lasting results; many find themselves back in old patterns.

It's because of long-term conditioning that they have experienced over the years that brings their behavior back to their former, less positive self.

In order to get more lasting results, you should write down the things you would like to do and the person you would like to be. Formulate a clear vision of things you want, whether it is health, money, relationships, career, and so forth. In order to change the outer self, you need to first change the inner self – the things that go on in your mind. You need a way to tell what type of inner self you have by reflecting on your life and the results you have been getting thus far.

What I also do to strengthen myself, as I mentioned earlier, is give myself positive affirmations by saying positive things about myself. Earlier, I mentioned that I constantly say, "*It is possible.*" Just by saying it repeatedly, it has changed my life for the better. I recommend it highly. Give yourself positive feedback, become aware when you are in a negative state, and refuse it. When you decide to choose positive thoughts, you will see that your self-image will change and become stronger than you ever thought possible.

My message to you:

1. Maintain a positive outlook and try to think positively always.

2. Remain strong, no matter what negative forces you meet.

3. Your thoughts create the reality you reside in.

4. Dust off all the negative thoughts you have of yourself and others.

5. Positive people help others who are in need of help.

6. Understand that negative people refrain from helping others.

7. Write down all the positive and negative thoughts you had during the day/week/month/year.

8. Write down what you are willing to do in order to change your way of thinking.

9. You always have a choice, so choose positive thoughts.

10. You can change what goes on outside by changing what goes on in your mind.

11. Never give up.

12. Reflect over your life and find your "why" – the reason you want to change.

13. Other people's negative thoughts and words do not have to become your reality.

14. Say "No" to all negativity and "Yes" to all that is positive.

15. Have a clear vision of what you want to do and who you want to become.
16. Give yourself positive feedback; say great things about yourself every day.
17. It is possible. You can do it.

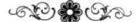

Chapter 4
Fear

Don't focus on the fear; instead, focus on the solution and you will see that there is nothing you cannot handle. I think fear is given too much space. So many people prevent themselves from changing their lives for the better because of fear. An African proverb says, "If there's no enemy within, then the enemy out there can't do me any harm."

Fear holds back many people; I've always wondered what prevents people from achieving their full potential and I have come to the conclusion after years of research on the subject that there are only two true fears: the fear of heights and unexpected loud noises. Everything else is something that you have created in your thoughts. We are capable of incredible things and, as I mentioned before, there is nothing in this world you can't handle.

It all depends on what you think, how you choose to direct what you think about, and how you view yourself. The more you choose to invest in yourself, the less you will fear – knowledge that has helped me tremendously. I am no longer afraid to go up on stage and speak in front of people, start a new business, lead and manage people, or take on a project that I have no experience in. I do get nervous now and then, but I'm no longer afraid, because I focus more on the solution rather than the fear itself. The more you believe in yourself, the less the fear can affect you.

There are three areas in which we may feel pain or fear. The first is fear of change, which makes many people afraid of losing something or getting into a situation that they have not previously experienced. People become afraid of losing something they like and care about, such as, *"If I make this change, I might lose my job, my partner, or a relationship with my friends."*

This reminds me of when I was working for a telecommunications company - one of the country's largest, in fact —I felt that I had reached the ceiling. There were no development opportunities for me. I wanted so much more and I knew that I was capable of so much more. I remember the fear generated from everyone when I told my friends about my plan to resign. They did not understand how or why one would resign from permanent employment. What would happen if I couldn't find a new job? What was I supposed to do then?

If I stayed there, at least I would have financial security by receiving monthly salary, but I knew that I wanted to evolve. I wanted to lead people, inspire people, and help people grow. I wanted to be a part of creating programs that would develop businesses and pursue new opportunities. I later resigned from my full-time employment; it may have been a tough period afterwards, but I eventually made it, and I'm happy that I decided to move on.

I remember being afraid of what the others had told me about the things that I would lose before I resigned from my job. For a while, it almost convinced me to remain at the company, but what made me finally resign was that I chose not to focus on what I would lose, but instead focused on what I had to gain.

What I have noticed when dealing with fear of change is that it makes people stay where they are because they focus on the thought *"What if?"* They put so much energy into stressing about every eventuality that it takes over and talks them in to staying put.

Another fear that we humans have is the fear of the process itself. *What will the journey be like? Where will I end up?* It reminds me of when I started a company and how the process scared me. There were so many questions that intimidated me, because I had no training in the field, I had no contacts, and I didn't have the money…how could it be done? I could have easily gone astray before ever starting the business.

Had I focused on my fears, they would have stopped me, but I chose to focus on the solution instead. It's okay if I don't know anything about the industry – I can always learn. It's okay that I do not have any contacts – I can always find out what type of contacts I need and acquire them. By taking that approach, my fears were minimized and I chose to start the business. I am very glad that I did, because of what I learned along the way, the contacts I did make, the amazing products and trips I have experienced, and all the people I got to lead and work with. I'm extremely grateful that I chose to take the plunge.

As I mentioned previously, the magic lies in seeing the positive instead of the negative, and that the process is not something negative, but something meaningful. It allows you to become the person you want to be.

The third fear we have is the end result: *What if things do not turn out as planned? What should I do with myself then? What if I do not succeed?* As in the previous example, it is vitally important to focus on the positive. In everything negative lies something positive; it's all about what you choose to focus on. I encourage you to think positively and to focus on the positive; you will soon see that you can take on challenges that you otherwise would not have accepted. Remember that fear is something that you have created all by yourself. It comes from your thoughts, so start thinking positively, start loving yourself, and begin seeing yourself for who you really are – a person with tremendous abilities.

My message to you:

1. Do not focus on the fear; instead, focus on the solution.
2. Take this proverb to heart; "If there's no enemy within, then the enemy out there can't do me any harm."
3. Do not let fear hold you back.
4. There is nothing in this world that you cannot handle.
5. The more you believe in yourself, the less you will fear.
6. Think not of what you might lose; think instead of what you might gain.
7. The magic lies in seeing the positive rather than the negative.

Chapter 5
Developing goals

How do you go about setting goals and why is it important to set goals? In this chapter, I will outline what a goal is and what goals need to contain in order for them to be powerful and useful. There are many who simply wander through life without ever setting any goals - and then you also have people who seem to get whatever they desire. The main reason that some people get what they want in life is because they have goals and they know where they are going. Goals are a vital ingredient for personal development. Having a goal is the same thing as having a clear vision for the future; life gets so much easier when you know where you are going, how long it will take, and what steps need to be taken in order to get there, rather than just wandering around every day, hoping to get lucky.

I often tell people that the reason so many people hate Mondays is because they don't have a goal set for themselves. After the weekend, Monday arrives and the anxiety sets in. Many people feel horrible because they are going back to jobs they hate. I used to be the type of person that hated Mondays; I still remember how I would feel when I laid in bed before it was time to get up and prepare for work. I never wanted to leave my bed - it was that horrible. However, things changed when I made a conscious and deliberate decision to begin enjoying my job. I took a sheet of paper and divided it into two columns. In the left column, I listed all the things I disliked about my job and in the right column, I listed all the things that I liked. At that time, I was in sales and my performance was less than ideal, which meant that I was not making the type of money of which I was capable. Therefore, I decided to focus more on the positive things about my job. I directed my thoughts away from anger at not making the type of money I wanted towards identifying areas for potential growth.

I decided that I would increase my sales within six months and I made a conscious decision to truly believe that I would achieve my goals. I told myself that I was not just an average salesperson; instead, I was one of the best, the type of salesman that is hard to find in the marketplace. I wrote down the salary I wanted and put it on my bathroom mirror, my fridge, and as the wallpaper on my computer screen. That way, I saw it often and was reminded of the task I had to accomplish. It was intimidating at first, as my mind wanted to initially hold me back when I wrote down the figure I wanted. I could feel how the negative thoughts came up instantly – *you really think you can do all that?*

The battle had begun. After writing down the desired amount, I started listing all the things I would do to achieve it. That list included everything from reading more books about sales to studying up on the business to get a better sense of our customers and why they wanted to have our products. I also decided that I would spend more time with my colleagues and share information on how we could present our information in a better way, as well as how we could become better at listening to what potential customers had to say. I also decided that I would not engage in anything else except behaviors and activities that would improve my performance. I reviewed my goal every day and monitored my performance, comparing daily, weekly, and monthly sales. I also knew that I had to change my attitude towards my profession; in other words, I had to love selling, listening, and talking to people. I had to basically change my entire perspective on selling. I was no longer going to sell; I was going to help people by bringing value to their life. That approach worked well for me and I started to gradually feel better about my profession, the company, and myself. It took a long time, but I became better at my job. My reason for doing all of this wasn't because I wanted more money; I knew that I could be the type of person who deliver great quality work, as well as a person who was always happy and encouraging. I had lost my way and had to find my way back to who I wanted to be.

I'm not saying that I am now the perfect salesperson. For instance, I later got another job as a salesperson, but I didn't perform well in that new position. I was simply not selling enough. I wanted to, but my heart wasn't aligned with that belief. I was aiming to become a supervisor, as I believed more in being a supervisor than a salesperson. Therefore, I didn't pour everything I had into becoming the best salesperson; I was simply selling because it was my job. The whole time, I was thinking about the supervisor position more than the selling, which is why I failed. I believe that everyone can be great at what they dedicate themselves to, but must of us are scattered. We want a thousand things at once, but if we could just focus on perfecting one craft, we could be unstoppable. I strongly recommend that if you want to achieve something, focus on one thing and do it well, rather than trying to do a thousand things at the same time.

A goal needs to be specific. There are those who have some idea of what they want to achieve, but for the most part, those ideas are vague visions. A great goal must be crystal clear. For instance, if I ask someone what their goal is, they might reply, "My goal is to buy a car". That goal is a vague vision in my opinion, because the moment they say they intend to buy a car, I start thinking of many different car manufacturers, different models, colors, sizes, and more. If a person said: I am going to get a car on the 15th of next month, a 2010 black Volvo XC90 with seven seats, a beige interior, 20-inch rims and a 220hp diesel engine that will cost X amount of dollars from X store. If a person said that instead, I would automatically paint a picture in my mind of that car – crystal clear.

I used a car as an example, but you can apply the same thought process to anything in life. A clear vision is easier to turn into reality, and it also allows you to stay focused on your journey. With a vague vision, you risk changes along the road and you end up with something you never wanted. **A goal needs to be big and compelling**, because the goal needs to excite you, motivate you, inspire you, and intimidate you. Your goals should allow you to grow by forcing you to create new approaches and find new ways of thinking. An idea that does not excite you will not help you grow, and the chances are good that you won't accomplish it - because it means nothing to you. In other words, aim high.

That sentiment makes me think about one of my childhood dreams. I always wanted to study at an American college, and growing up, I remember spending a lot of time thinking and fantasizing about the day I would receive my acceptance letter and how happy I would be. The joy of just the thought of being accepted literally brought tears to my eyes…I wanted it so badly. I never knew why and still don't. I didn't immediately apply after graduating gymnasium (equivalent to high school in the United States); in fact, I joined the military. After graduating from the military, I decided that I wanted to go back to school and get more training in business. However, this time around, I wanted my studies to be in the states. It was a very intimidating thought for me, particularly because of my worries of communicating and working in academic-level English. I spent a year working and studied English by myself in my spare time. I studied every word in the dictionary from A - Z and listened to radio shows that hardly played any music. I was studying and writing every day, even writing poems, which I think were quite good. I even wrote one in America that was dedicated to Mia; I called it „The Boy at the Window." Mia was in still in her last year of high school at that time. She always said that she and her older sister cried when they read the poem, and I still think of it as my best work so far. My concern at not comprehending academic English never left me while I was home in Sweden. Then came the day that I got home from work and opened the front door to find a large envelope on the floor. When I picked it up, I could see all the stamps and a mixed feeling of joy and fear ran through me. I opened the envelope and read the papers, which stated - *Dear Mr. Sassi, we are proud to announce that you have been accepted…* I was so overjoyed that I have no way to describe the feeling - my dream was finally coming true.

I eventually moved to San Francisco and got the chance to study at an American college; it was truly an experience that I will never forget.

A goal must be written down. This simple rule reminds me of the time I received an offer to become an investor in a business. A friend of mine had recommended me and asked if I could meet with the management to go through the business and the mission. I replied that I would be happy to meet with them. I knew the market they operated in, so I had some sense of how the business was structured and how it operated. It took several hours to get to their office, as I had to travel a long distance to a different town far from Gothenburg, where I lived at the time. When I got to the meeting, everyone greeted me very professionally and we eventually sat down to go through the businesses and discuss my involvement. I asked the CEO to show me the business plan, to which he replied that he could tell me everything about it. I repeated that I wanted to see the written documents, but he said that they didn't have any and that it was not necessary. He stated that he had everything in his mind. I had to turn them down because I can't rely on one man's memory. That approach is too vague; I consider myself flexible, but that was no way to run a business. One important aspect of growth comes from reflection and re-evaluation; they would miss a lot of useful information by not documenting anything. I had to turn around and travel all the way back home to Gothenburg. I wasn't angry or frustrated, because I learned something critical from that experience.

It is essential to write down everything, because as you write it down, the brain registers the activity for a second time. The act of writing enhances the memory of the topic; furthermore, it's useful to have it written down so that you can review the goal often. We all tend to get sidetracked sooner or later, so having things written down helps us find our way back. For example, I carry small pieces of paper with my goal written down so that I can review it daily.

A goal needs to be reviewed often. I mentioned earlier that reviewing goals helps us find our way back when we get sidetracked. I also want to emphasize that the depth of our sidetracks depends heavily on how often we review our goals. If you review your goals daily, or many times each day, the chances of being sidetracked are much smaller than for people who review their goals monthly or even yearly. Being reminded of what you need to focus on is vital; the more you remind yourself, the more likely you are to remain on track and achieve your goals.

A goal needs to be aligned with your own beliefs; if it closely aligns with your core beliefs, then you won't need to put much effort into convincing yourself to move towards your dream. Your goal will already be a part of you - something you already represent. You won't be as easily tempted by other distractions if your goal aligns with your beliefs.

A goal needs to have a strategy. It is important to develop a game plan for how you intend to achieve your goal. Don't worry if you have no clue; it will eventually come to you. There are steps you need to take, but there is always a way. Everything will come to you in time, particularly because not knowing will spark innovative thinking. You will start to think differently and seek out people you normally wouldn't, which means creating new relationships. One way to create a strategy is by answering the following questions: *Why? How? Where? When? Whom?* Your questions could be, for instance: Why am I doing this? How is it going to be carried out? Where will it be carried out? When is it going to be carried out? By whom or for whom is it being carried out? Practice asking yourself questions with these five W's and you'll set yourself up for far greater success in terms of achieving your goal.

A goal needs to be measurable. The reason that goals must be measurable is because it gives you clarity on how the process is going and you'll be able to accurately track your progress. Many people say that a goal should be realistic and attainable, but I would say that you should simply aim for what you desire. Just because one person or a group doesn't believe something is possible doesn't mean that you can't achieve it. People throughout history have overcome obstacles and achieved dreams and goals that have seemed impossible to other people. I urge you to go for your dreams and goals, regardless of what people tell you. Just remember to track and record your progress so that you know how far you have to go until you reach those goals.

A goal needs to be divided into smaller parts. In order to make the journey much easier, break your goal down into smaller parts because smaller targets are easier to accomplish. Those accomplishments will give you more confidence, increase your determination, and give you the necessary energy to take on the next target. You can celebrate and pat yourself on the back more often, whereas one big goal has a greater chance of exhausting you and often takes more time to accomplish, which only gives those negative thoughts time to come back and start haunting you, telling you that you've invested so much time and energy without results. However, with smaller goals, you get to see your progress, which ultimately adds up to your one major goal.

There must be a strong reason for why you want to achieve the goal. This is the key element, in my opinion. You must have a real reason why you want to get up and fight, because life will knock you down over and over again. Your reason, your "why," will be what encourages you to get back on your feet and continue to fight. You will face setbacks, you will want to quit, people will fail you, and all hell will break loose before life lets you win. At some point, you will probably want to give in and do something else, but your reason will be the force that keeps you alive and moving forward. Before your start marching towards your dream, make sure you know why you're heading in that direction — that knowledge just might save your life.

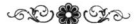

Chapter 6
Money

Money is one of the key factors that drives
the world engine and is something I believe
that all people would like to have more of.
This is because I believe that having more
money gives you more choices; you will no
longer be limited to certain activities. If a
business opportunity presents itself, you are
more likely to invest if you have enough
funds or know how to acquire the necessary
funds to start that business. It's possible to
start a business with no money down; I have
done it and believe that it is possible for you
to also start with nothing.

A lot of people have done it and so can you. Money is not something I have always mastered. In fact, I have been in heavy debt, and I've been broke to the point where I couldn't see a way out, but as you have read, I came to a point where I got sick and tired of being sick and tired. I had to do something about it and I told myself that I would never be in that position again.

Money is a tool and it's important that you learn to master it. My team and I have developed a system at marcussassi.com that will help you master money and have it work for you. I always tell my friends that if you have some money and you don't need it, remember that there is always someone out there who needs the money. You can either give it away or employ somebody that will bring value to you with that money.

I have found through meeting people and doing research that the wealthiest people behave like poor people, while poor people try to behave as if they are wealthy. Poor people have come to be fond of consumerism and most of them don't manage their money well. They live paycheck-to-paycheck and if you visit their home, you'll often find that they have collected a lot of stuff - many of their homes are filled with possessions.

I'm not saying that this is a wrong way to live life; everyone is entitled to whatever lifestyle suits them, but if you spend time with someone that is financially well off, you'll find out that almost every one of them is also fond of consumerism, but a different *kind* of consumerism. Instead of buying "stuff," they buy financial products, such as dividend-yielding stocks, bonds, etc. They also manage their money well, which is the underlying difference, and it gives them the perspective they need.

I strongly believe that you can become financial wealthy by being an employee, but that requires the discipline to follow through on your goal of achieving financial freedom and also investing. Saving will take you far, but investing will take you further. I didn't have anyone teach me about money; I had to learn about it the hard way and I've made huge mistakes. At times, I have spent all I had and much more. I wish that I had had someone to teach me and show me how it all works. I don't want you to make the same mistakes that I made. You don't have to continue making mistakes in handling money; that's why my team and I have worked hard to build a management and educational system that will teach you everything about money, because life becomes so much easier. Trust me – you will be able to sleep better at night and not always be anxious or scared about the future.

I know a lot of people who would be in a whole lot of stress if they lost their job today; they would need to start working at a new job immediately just to stay afloat. I don't want you to live like that; it's not a healthy life. I'm telling you this because I have experienced it first hand and it's not something that I recommend.

Writing this makes me think back to when I was un-employed and wasn't receiving anything from the social program for unemployment. I was out of work for six months, but luckily I had some money saved away. It was not much, however, and those funds ran out very quickly, leaving me totally out of money. I had no money to pay for my apartment, electricity, or even food. I had to go to my friend's house to eat because I had nothing. I will never forget it. I couldn't sleep for days and I lost a lot of weight. I remember that whenever I saw the mailman come toward my apartment, I almost had a breakdown, because he never came with any good news. He only came to deliver more bad news for me – the bills he carried… the bills I couldn't afford to pay.

After a while, I got a phone call from a debt collector, and that was the tipping point for me. I remember that I sat on the floor and cried because I had no money to pay my bills. While crying, something in me happened. I stopped crying and firmly told myself that this would be the last time I got in this position.

I needed a change and I was willing to do anything to get out of my current living situation. Luckily, I got my-self a job and although it took me many months to get back on track, I did. I also began to monitor and record my finances, making sure that I didn't spend more than I earned. Most of my monthly salary went to paying off my debts. I made sure to pay more than what the debt collector billed me every month so that the debt would decrease faster than expected.

I started to save all my receipts so that I could see how much various categories cost me each month, which helped me change my behavior. It was painful, but I did it. The desire to get out debt was strong enough that it kept me on track and kept me going forward. I stayed with the same plan after I got out of debt as well; I would imagine that I was still in debt, even when I was debt-free. However, instead of paying off the debt, I would pay myself. I opened a bank account in another bank and started saving.

The first step was to save up for small emergencies, which was $1000 dollars. When I was done with that, I began saving for medium-range emergencies, which is approximately 6 months' worth of salary. Finally, when that was done, I saved up for major emergencies, which was 12 months' worth of salary. It took me a very long time to accumulate all the accounts, but I did it. I'm so happy that I did, and I strongly believe that you can too. I didn't have a high-paying job, not even an average paying job, for that matter.

After accumulating all the savings, I started to invest part of my salary, and I began by buying dividend-yielding stocks. I kept doing this month after month. After a while, I became better at saving, I knew what I was spending money on, and I knew all the accounts in the back of my head. When I had saved enough money, I finally knew that I could start my own business. Everything takes time. I find that a lot of people are intimidated by how much time some things take, but whatever you do, don't stop. Just keep moving forward month after month and you will eventually find yourself reaching your financial goals. I strongly believe that anyone can do it.

Creating financial wealth is actually very simple. What's hard, however, is fighting the temptations all around us. That is where many of us fail, so work on your discipline and your thoughts, in addition to reviewing your goals every day so you don't get sidetracked. Remember that you deserve to live a more prosperous life. You can do it if you're willing to raise your standards and use that willpower of yours.

Think about all the people that will reach the age of sixty-five without any savings or financial education. That's not a life that you want for yourself and I believe that those who are in that position don't want to be where they are either. You can change your future; it's never too late. You simply need to get started investing in yourself. Convince yourself that you are going to make a better life for yourself and those you care about, develop a game plan, and make it a reality. You don't need to experience the pain of heavy financial burden. I would recommend that you don't fixate on earning more money – do more with what you have.

The most important thing is not what you make; it is what you keep. The amount you keep is what will create a difference in your life, so start monitoring all your expenses and see what you can change about your purchasing behavior. No matter how impossible it seems, we can all afford to make adjustments.

Don't forget to reward yourself along the journey, either. It's no fun to only save and invest month in and month out. That process will be far too painful if you never get to reward yourself.

My message to you:

1. Money is a tool that gives you more choices to choose from.
2. Money can be mastered, so have it work for you instead of working for it.
3. Get out of debt and stay debt-free.
4. Saving can get you far, but investing will get you further.
5. Poor people buy products; wealthy people buy financial products.
6. Invest in your financial education. (www.marcussassi.com)
7. Monitor all your expenses. (www.marcussassi.com)
8. Do not spend more than you earn.
9. Save all receipts.

10. Save short-term financial emergency funds.

11. Save mid-term financial emergency funds.

12. Save long-term financial emergency funds.

13. Everyone can achieve financial freedom.

14. Be persistent in your savings and investments.

15. If you are in debt, pay more than you are being billed.

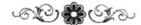

Chapter 7

Commitment

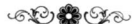

Commitment is stronger than desire. Commitment actually means that you are going to keep whatever promises you have made. You execute them and continue true to your own integrity.

It's all about being loyal to your responsibilities. I strongly hope that after you have read this book, you will be committed to grow and do whatever it takes to improve your life.

It's much easier when you have a strong self-belief, mental strength, and have developed the skill of developing goals. What I have offered you is the foundation upon which commitment can be built.

You need to be committed because you will en-counter obstacles – everyone does. You will en-counter obstacles too, and when you do, being committed will save you, because you will not give up. Instead, you will say to yourself, "*Okay, now how do I solve this,*" and you will work toward solving it.

It doesn't matter what field you're in; commitment applies to all fields. If my wife and I hadn't been committed to our relationship, we would have never been together for more than ten years. If Bill Gates was not committed, Microsoft would not be the company we have come to know and respect. If I was not committed to my dreams, then I wouldn't have begun my journey to empower people.

I have worked and spent time with a lot people and I have been hurt many times. This is because I couldn't see the difference between a promise and being committed. I've always strived for commitment, even when I didn't know what it meant. People said that they would show up or execute a certain task that I had given them, but what they gave me was a promise, not a commitment. When someone is committed, they are invested in something; they are attached or in tune with it psychologically, which means that they will do whatever it takes to execute that task. They will not bow down, no matter what they en-counter and they will not change the plan. They will work until it's done. That is the sign of commitment; they are simply dedicated.

A promise, however, is something that can change, just like strategies change dependent on inner or outer factors. Therefore, be committed and be serious about the health of your life. Look for ways to make it happen, because everything is possible if you want it to be.

Being committed is all about the process. I tell you this because in life, we get the things we want for who we are. I want you to become a person that is able to take action and actually follow through on whatever goal or dream you have set for yourself.

I'm committed to help you become that person, which is why I've done everything in my power with this book, the action planner, and marcussassi.com. If you work through the process, then there's no limit to what you can do for yourself and the people you care about most.

My message to you:
1. Commitment means keeping whatever promise you made, doing whatever it takes to execute it, and remaining true to your own integrity.
2. It is easier to be committed with strong self-belief, mental strength, and goal-setting skills.
3. Being committed will be one of the factors that will get you back on track when you feel sidetracked or lost.

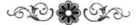

Chapter 8
Attitude

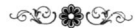

I could have gotten mad when I didn't get
the job as a portfolio manager, or that other
time when I didn't get the job as a supervisor, or when I was turned down because of
my skin color. I could have gotten mad, but
I didn't. I didn't let that negative voice in my
head talk me down. I fought it and won. I
believed that I had greatness in me and that
one day it would be my turn. Sure, I've been
down many times - there's nothing wrong
with being down. The key is not to stay there
for long. Don't let failure become a part of
you.

I used to get mad when things didn't go my way. I would spend days, weeks, or even months just thinking about it, but that never gave me anything of value. At least, not until I changed my attitude toward life and the experiences that life had to offer. Now, my viewpoint is that I always have a choice; I can either be mad or happy.

I try to always, think, speak, walk, and dress in a positive manner and spend time with positive and encouraging people. I've found that it gets me closer to whatever I want far easier than embracing a negative outlook. So what is attitude? I would say that attitude is how you choose to see the world – the lens you use to filter the world – and it can either be positive or negative.

Some people are negative toward the rain, while others see it as a positive thing. For instance, some think about the fact that they get wet, while someone else might think about rain being good for trees and crops. Life is all about your perspective of things. It's important to understand that you can adjust your attitude toward life. It's entirely possible, and you have the choice to do it.

The key elements to changing your attitude include being aware that it's all about choice and that you must sincerely foster a positive attitude. You also need to understand that changing your attitude takes time, so you need to stay positive as often as possible. Attitude is a habit and habits take time to settle in and become a part of you.

If you feel great mentally, emotionally, physically, and spiritually, then you will have a much easier path toward changing your attitude.

You may feel like it's impossible, but I believe you can. Like all the topics in this book, you can change anything negative into something positive. If you want to have a more positive outlook in your life, then you need to be determined that change can and will happen. You can do this by creating a vision board and list constructive and positive solutions, while always working on strengthening your will power.

We humans tend to travel between darkness and light, smiles and frowns.

I've found that to live in a positive manner, one must be grateful. I tell myself every day what I'm grateful for. For example, I'm grateful for being alive, having my health, my wife, my daughter, my friends, and the ability to help other people.

When I say that I'm grateful, it's like peace crawls into my heart so that I am no longer frustrated or irritated about things when something negative happens.

Start being grateful and try to stay positive as often as you can. Soon, you'll start to see that the way you view the world has changed. Start loving yourself - and everything about yourself. Be open and humble and understand that there's nothing in life that you cannot do. If you have something about yourself that you want to change, you can do it. For instance, if you get upset quickly, you can easily change that behavior if you're willing to do the work by investing yourself.

To love yourself is a vital personality aspect and it helps when creating a stronger sense of self-belief and a positive attitude toward yourself and everything else in life. Be humble and treat others just the way you yourself would like to be treated. The key areas to work on are your mental, physical, emotional, and spiritual self.

My message to you:

1. Attitude is a choice; you can to choose to be either happy or sad.

2. Changing attitudes takes time, which requires that you remain persistent.

3. It is possible to change your attitude, but you must sincerely want to change if a change is to come.

4. It is easier to change your attitude when you feel great mentally, emotionally, physically, and spiritually. Work on the areas that you feel need more work.

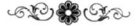

Chapter 9

Encouraging friends

I want you to know that not everyone will
cheer for you, help you, or be there for you.
You need to accept that fact. I don't want you
to start naturally disliking people, but you
need to know that reaching your dreams and
goals can be a very lonely road. It sometimes
happens that people no longer want to spend
time with you out of envy or hatred. However, understand that they don't actually hate
you; they simply have not found their own
path yet. People who can't see something for
themselves can't see it for others.

If you find yourself feeling lonely, don't get mad or frustrated, just be grateful that you have been blessed to find your way. Understand that your friends may not always help you, but there are people out there who share your vision and who would like to team up with you or give you a helping hand. It's crucial that you start finding those people, because you can go far by yourself, but much further with the help of people who see your potential and share your core beliefs.

I myself would not be where I am right now if it were not due to my own self-belief, the loving support of my wife Mia, my team, who believes in me, the work we do, and in themselves, and never forgetting my friends that motivated me to seek my dreams. It's vitally important that you find people who will be there for you and cheer for you on your journey. It's possible that you might not find those people within your friends; you may need to look elsewhere, such as network groups, mentorships, etc. We cannot do everything by ourselves; we all need help at times. That's why the most successful people emphasize on building great teams.

I encourage you to surround yourself with encouraging people that will support you, experience joy with you, motivate and inspire you and give you that energy boost to get in touch with other people that are able to help you grow.

My message to you:

1. Not everyone is going to be there for you.
2. It is vitally important that you find people who will cheer you on and help you grow.

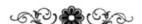

Action planner

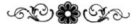

Who are you today?

_____

_____

_____

_____

_____

_____

_____

_____

_____

_____

_____

_____

_____

_____

Who do you want to become?

_____

_____

_____

_____

_____

_____

_____

_____

_____

_____

_____

_____

_____

What would you most love to do?

What I would love to do	This has stopped me
1 .	
2	
3	
4	
5	
6	
7	

List your weaknesses

_____

_____

_____

_____

_____

_____

_____

_____

_____

_____

_____

_____

_____

_____

What steps will you take to diminish your weakness?

_____

_____

_____

_____

_____

_____

_____

_____

_____

_____

_____

_____

_____

_____

List your strengths

_____

_____

_____

_____

_____

_____

_____

_____

_____

_____

_____

_____

What steps will you take to improve your strengths?

_____

_____

_____

_____

_____

_____

_____

_____

_____

_____

_____

_____

_____

What is your vision for your health?

_____

_____

_____

_____

_____

_____

_____

_____

_____

_____

_____

_____

What steps will you take to turn your vision for your health into a reality?

_____

_____

_____

_____

_____

_____

_____

_____

_____

_____

_____

_____

_____

_____

What is your vision for your relationship with your wife/
husband?

_____

_____

_____

_____

_____

_____

_____

_____

_____

_____

_____

_____

_____

What steps will you take to turn your vision for your relationship into a reality?

_____

_____

_____

_____

_____

_____

_____

_____

_____

_____

_____

_____

_____

What is your vision for your finances?

_____

_____

_____

_____

_____

_____

_____

_____

_____

_____

_____

_____

_____

What steps will you take to turn your vision for your finances into a reality?

_____

_____

_____

_____

_____

_____

_____

_____

_____

_____

_____

_____

What is your vision for your career?

_____

_____

_____

_____

_____

_____

_____

_____

_____

_____

_____

_____

_____

What steps will you take to turn your vision for your career into a reality?

_____

_____

_____

_____

_____

_____

_____

_____

_____

_____

_____

_____

_____

What is your vision for your business?

_____

_____

_____

_____

_____

_____

_____

_____

_____

_____

_____

_____

_____

What steps will you take to turn your vision for your business into a reality?

_____

_____

_____

_____

_____

_____

_____

_____

_____

_____

_____

_____

What is your vision for your family?

_____

_____

_____

_____

_____

_____

_____

_____

_____

_____

_____

_____

What steps will you take to turn your vision for your family into a reality?

_____

_____

_____

_____

_____

_____

_____

_____

_____

_____

_____

_____

_____

What is your vision for your spirituality?

_____

_____

_____

_____

_____

_____

_____

_____

_____

_____

_____

_____

What steps will you take to turn your vision for your
spirituality into a reality?

_____

_____

_____

_____

_____

_____

_____

_____

_____

_____

_____

_____

About the author

Marcus Sassi is best known for his motivation and drive as an entrepreneur with many years of experience running businesses. He has also been a business consultant, helping other entrepreneurs start and develop their own businesses.

Marcus lives in Gothenburg, Sweden with his wife Mia and daughter Leona. He enjoys reading, writing, mentoring, consulting with entrepreneurs, and spending quality time with his wife and daughter.

To learn more, visit the website at *www.marcussassi.com*

Marcus Sassi delivers the powerful strategies and techniques detailed in ***Ready to Take Action***
to companies and individuals.

For information on speaking events, corporate coaching, seminars, and workshops, contact Marcus at:

Marcus Sassi
www.marcussassi.com

WWW.MARCUSSASSI.COM